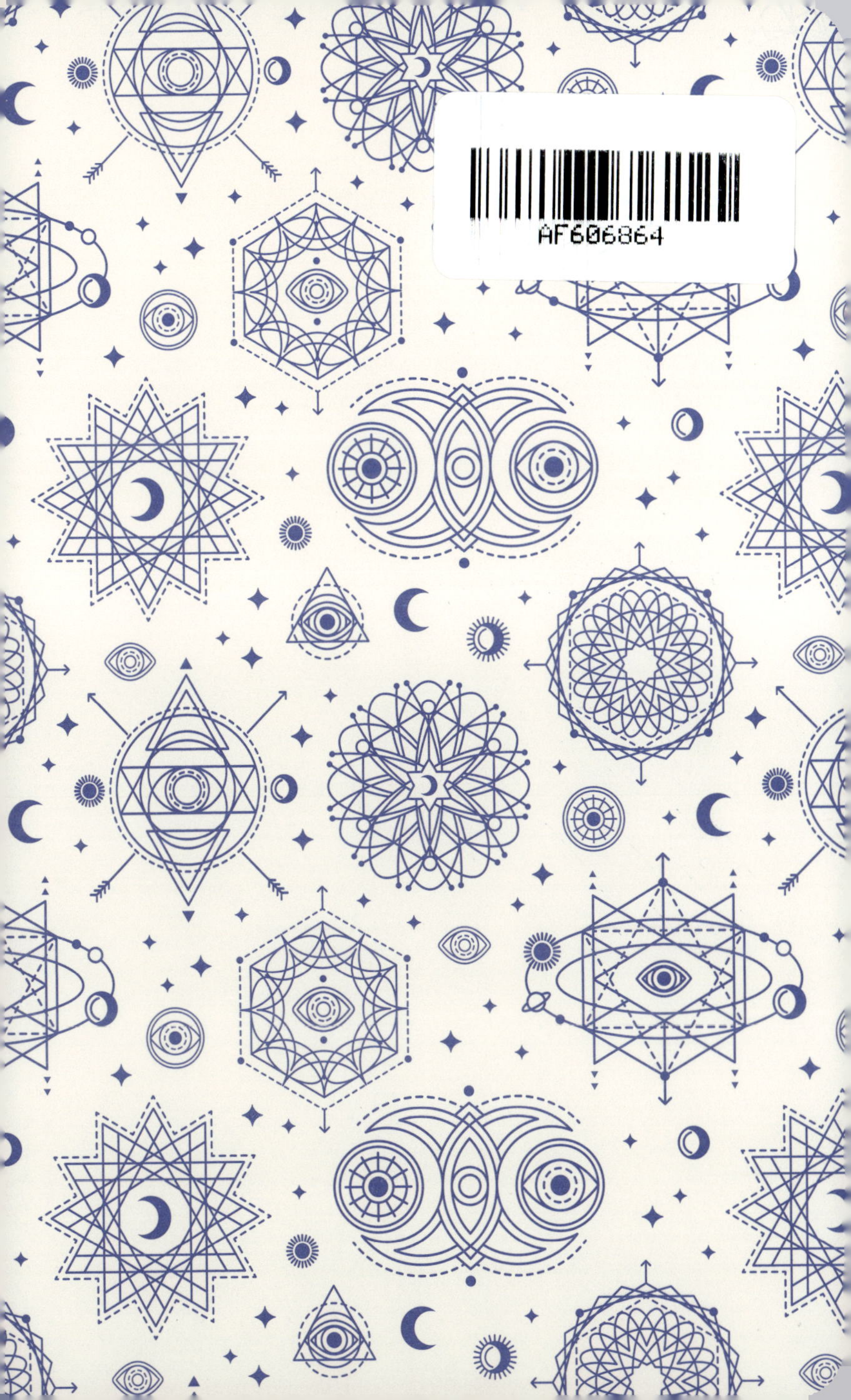
AF606864

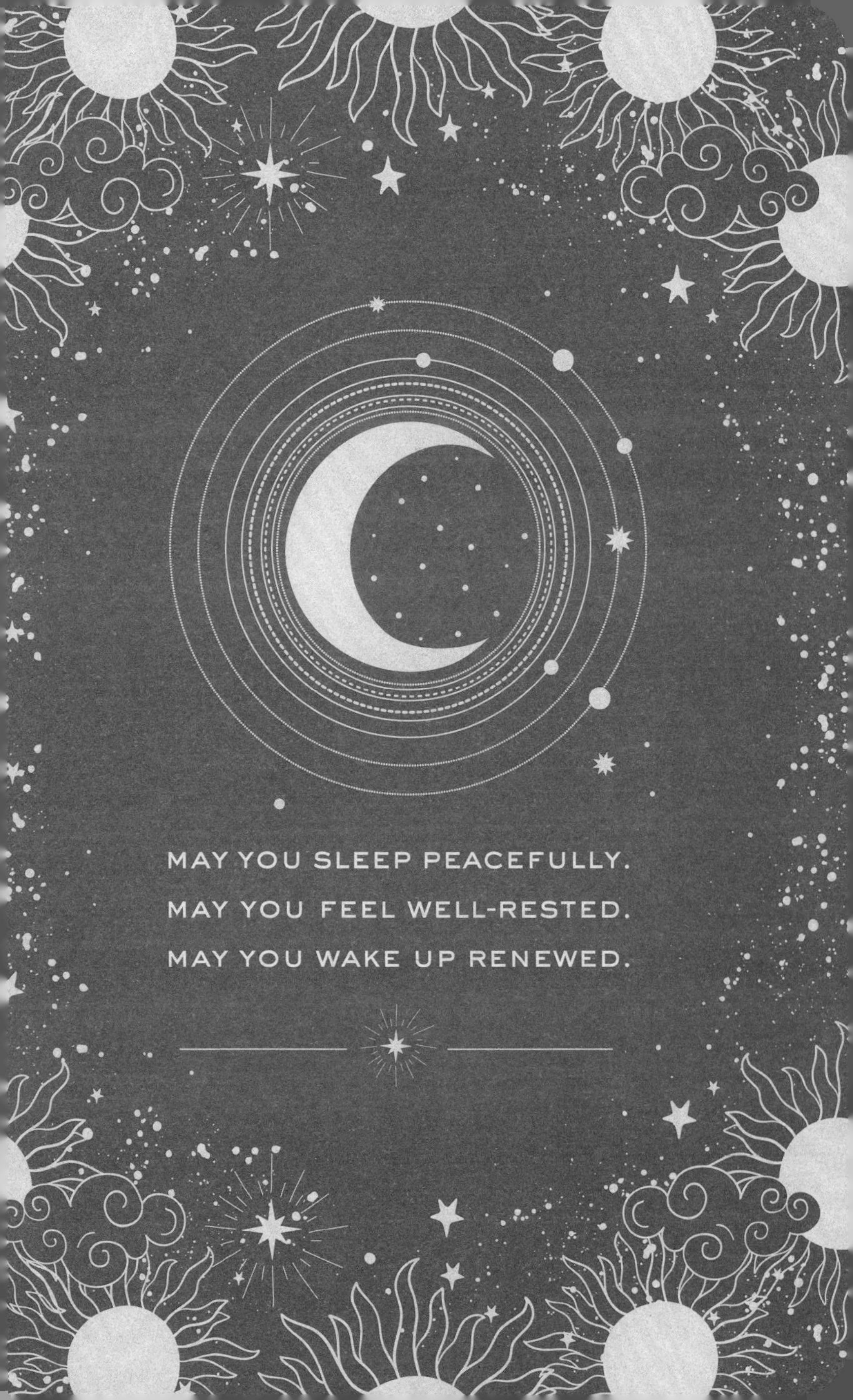
MAY YOU SLEEP PEACEFULLY.
MAY YOU FEEL WELL-RESTED.
MAY YOU WAKE UP RENEWED.

SLEEP IS ESSENTIAL TO YOUR PHYSICAL and mental health and maintaining healthy sleep habits is key to both the quality and quantity of sleep you can achieve.

How you manage stress can play a significant role in your ability to fall and stay asleep; and crafting a pre-bedtime routine that helps you unwind and signals to the body that sleep is approaching is essential to promote restful sleep. One of the best ways to de-stress and resolve your worries or concerns before bedtime is to write down what's on your mind and then set it aside for tomorrow.

This journal is a place to let your worries, thoughts, to-dos, or anything else in the corners of your mind rest. When your mind is clear and light, you will be able to invite rejuvenating sleep in.

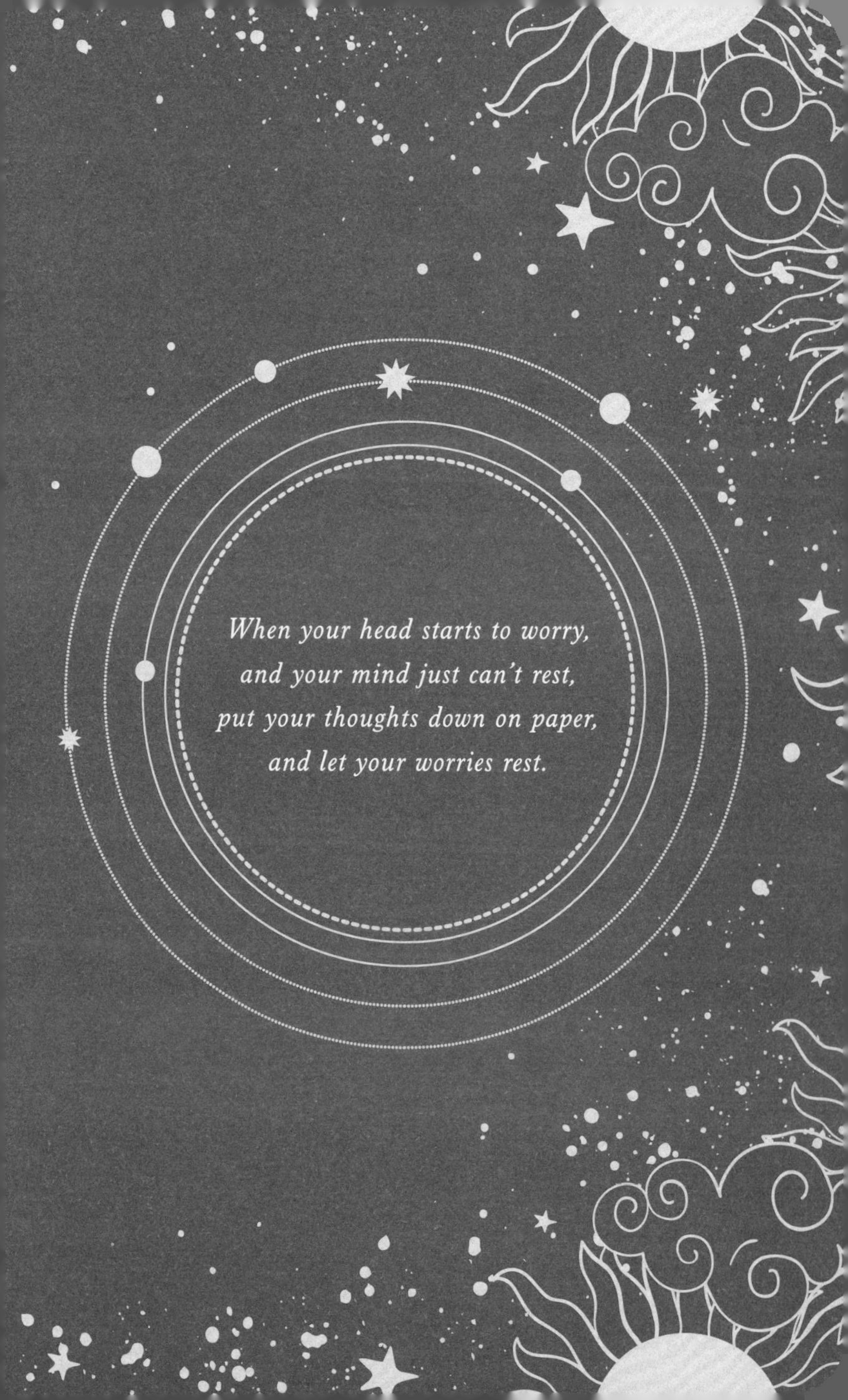
When your head starts to worry,
and your mind just can't rest,
put your thoughts down on paper,
and let your worries rest.

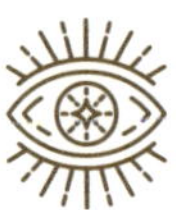

RUMINATING THOUGHTS

to clear from your mind

A RESTFUL MANTRA

to carry you to sleep

TAKE TIME TO PAUSE

"Put your thoughts to sleep, do not let them cast a shadow over the moon of your heart. Let go of thinking." —*Rumi*

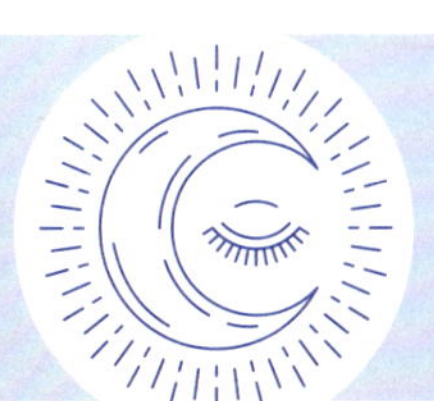

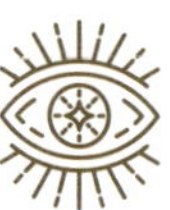

RUMINATING THOUGHTS

to clear from your mind

A RESTFUL MANTRA

to carry you to sleep

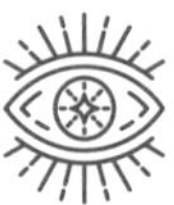

RUMINATING THOUGHTS

to clear from your mind

A RESTFUL MANTRA

to carry you to sleep

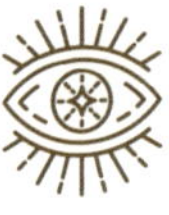

RUMINATING THOUGHTS

to clear from your mind

A RESTFUL MANTRA

to carry you to sleep

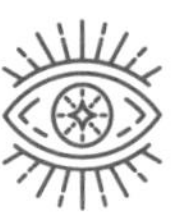

RUMINATING THOUGHTS

to clear from your mind

A RESTFUL MANTRA

to carry you to sleep

RUMINATING THOUGHTS

to clear from your mind

A RESTFUL MANTRA

to carry you to sleep

RUMINATING THOUGHTS

to clear from your mind

A RESTFUL MANTRA

to carry you to sleep

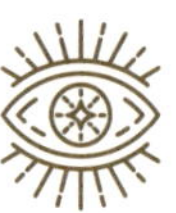

RUMINATING THOUGHTS

to clear from your mind

A RESTFUL MANTRA

to carry you to sleep

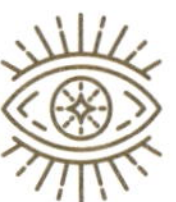

RUMINATING THOUGHTS

to clear from your mind

A RESTFUL MANTRA

to carry you to sleep

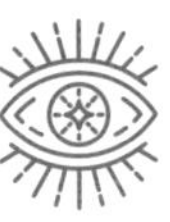

RUMINATING THOUGHTS

to clear from your mind

A RESTFUL MANTRA

to carry you to sleep

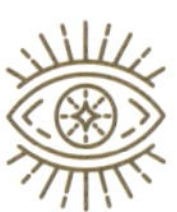

RUMINATING THOUGHTS

to clear from your mind

A RESTFUL MANTRA

to carry you to sleep

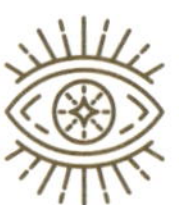

RUMINATING THOUGHTS

to clear from your mind

A RESTFUL MANTRA

to carry you to sleep

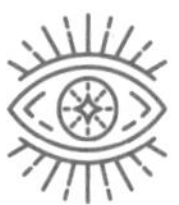

RUMINATING THOUGHTS

to clear from your mind

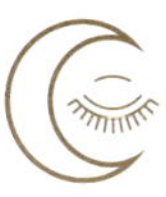

A RESTFUL MANTRA

to carry you to sleep

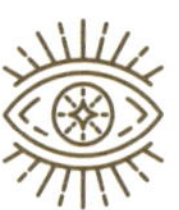

RUMINATING THOUGHTS

to clear from your mind

A RESTFUL MANTRA

to carry you to sleep

FIND COMFORT IN PEACE

"The best bed that a man can sleep on is peace." —*Somali proverb*

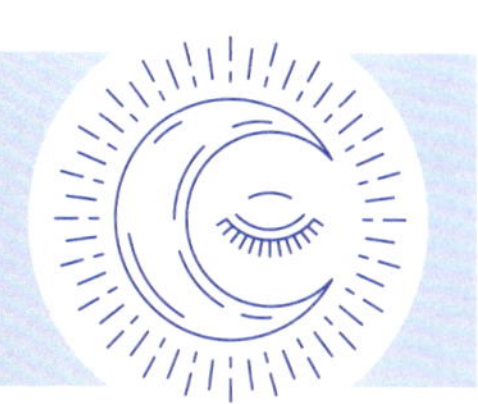

RUMINATING THOUGHTS

to clear from your mind

A RESTFUL MANTRA

to carry you to sleep

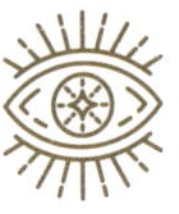

RUMINATING THOUGHTS

to clear from your mind

A RESTFUL MANTRA

to carry you to sleep

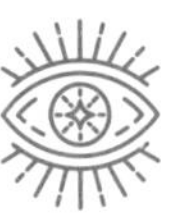

RUMINATING THOUGHTS

to clear from your mind

A RESTFUL MANTRA

to carry you to sleep

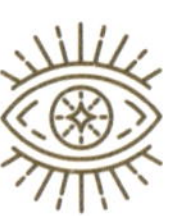

RUMINATING THOUGHTS

to clear from your mind

A RESTFUL MANTRA

to carry you to sleep

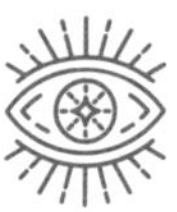

RUMINATING THOUGHTS

to clear from your mind

A RESTFUL MANTRA

to carry you to sleep

RUMINATING THOUGHTS

to clear from your mind

A RESTFUL MANTRA

to carry you to sleep

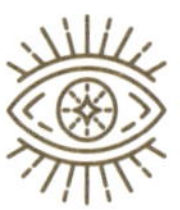

RUMINATING THOUGHTS

to clear from your mind

A RESTFUL MANTRA

to carry you to sleep

RUMINATING THOUGHTS

to clear from your mind

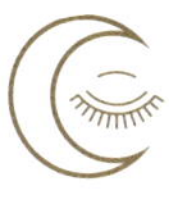

A RESTFUL MANTRA

to carry you to sleep

RUMINATING THOUGHTS

to clear from your mind

A RESTFUL MANTRA

to carry you to sleep

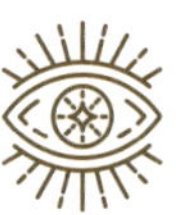

RUMINATING THOUGHTS

to clear from your mind

A RESTFUL MANTRA

to carry you to sleep

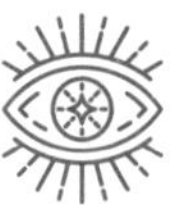

RUMINATING THOUGHTS

to clear from your mind

A RESTFUL MANTRA

to carry you to sleep

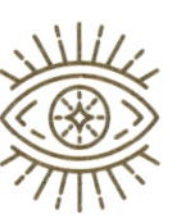

RUMINATING THOUGHTS

to clear from your mind

A RESTFUL MANTRA

to carry you to sleep

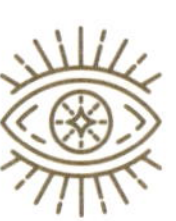

RUMINATING THOUGHTS

to clear from your mind

A RESTFUL MANTRA

to carry you to sleep

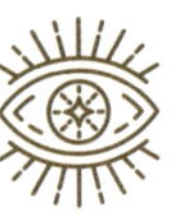

RUMINATING THOUGHTS

to clear from your mind

A RESTFUL MANTRA

to carry you to sleep

KNOW THAT YOU ARE SAFE

"When you lie down, you will not be afraid. Your sleep will be sweet." —*Proverbs 3:24*

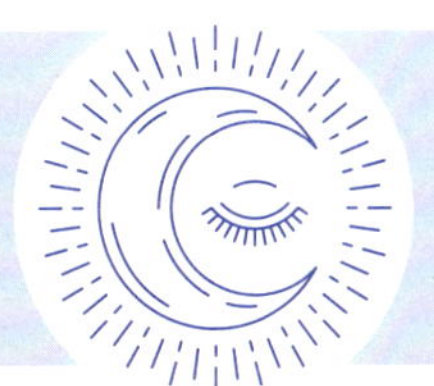

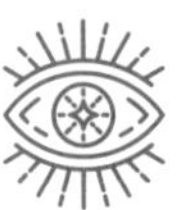

RUMINATING THOUGHTS

to clear from your mind

A RESTFUL MANTRA

to carry you to sleep

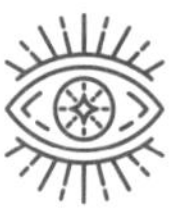

RUMINATING THOUGHTS

to clear from your mind

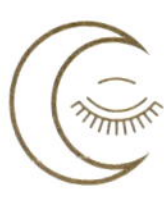

A RESTFUL MANTRA

to carry you to sleep

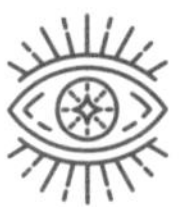

RUMINATING THOUGHTS

to clear from your mind

A RESTFUL MANTRA

to carry you to sleep

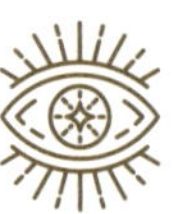

RUMINATING THOUGHTS

to clear from your mind

A RESTFUL MANTRA

to carry you to sleep

RUMINATING THOUGHTS

to clear from your mind

A RESTFUL MANTRA

to carry you to sleep

RUMINATING THOUGHTS

to clear from your mind

A RESTFUL MANTRA

to carry you to sleep

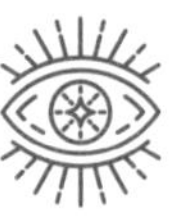

RUMINATING THOUGHTS

to clear from your mind

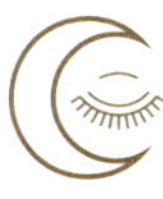

A RESTFUL MANTRA

to carry you to sleep

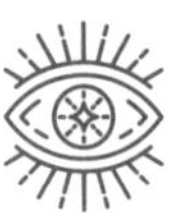

RUMINATING THOUGHTS

to clear from your mind

A RESTFUL MANTRA

to carry you to sleep

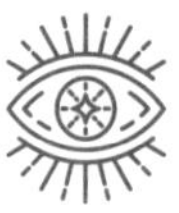

RUMINATING THOUGHTS

to clear from your mind

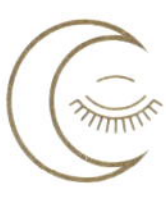

A RESTFUL MANTRA

to carry you to sleep

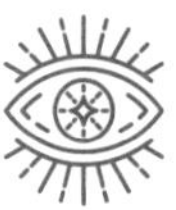

RUMINATING THOUGHTS

to clear from your mind

A RESTFUL MANTRA

to carry you to sleep

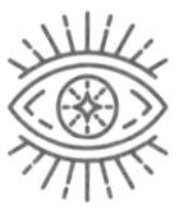

RUMINATING THOUGHTS

to clear from your mind

A RESTFUL MANTRA

to carry you to sleep

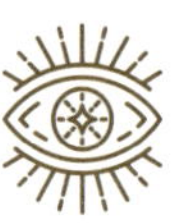

RUMINATING THOUGHTS

to clear from your mind

A RESTFUL MANTRA

to carry you to sleep

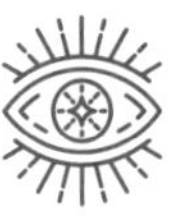

RUMINATING THOUGHTS

to clear from your mind

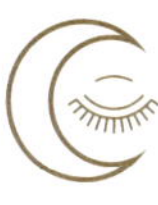

A RESTFUL MANTRA

to carry you to sleep

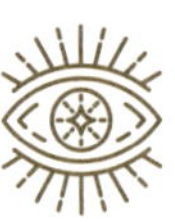

RUMINATING THOUGHTS

to clear from your mind

A RESTFUL MANTRA

to carry you to sleep

WELCOME YOUR DREAMS

"Your future depends on your dreams, so go to sleep." —*Mesut Barazany*

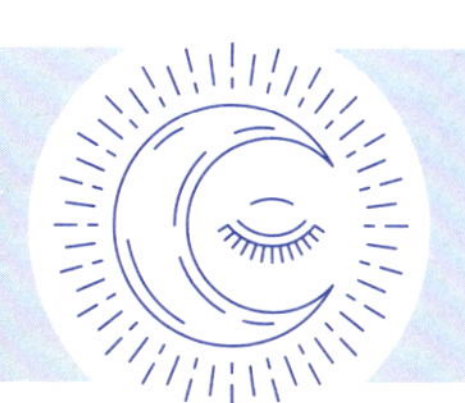

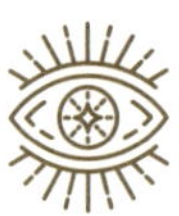

RUMINATING THOUGHTS

to clear from your mind

A RESTFUL MANTRA

to carry you to sleep

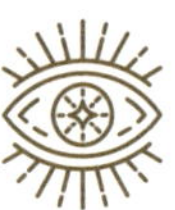

RUMINATING THOUGHTS

to clear from your mind

A RESTFUL MANTRA

to carry you to sleep

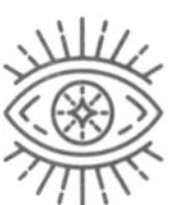

RUMINATING THOUGHTS

to clear from your mind

A RESTFUL MANTRA

to carry you to sleep

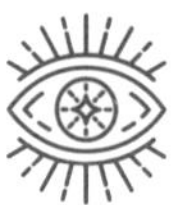

RUMINATING THOUGHTS

to clear from your mind

A RESTFUL MANTRA

to carry you to sleep

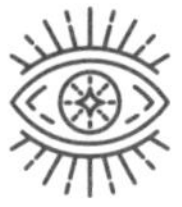

RUMINATING THOUGHTS

to clear from your mind

A RESTFUL MANTRA

to carry you to sleep

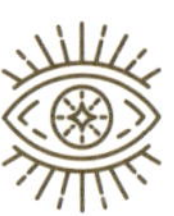

RUMINATING THOUGHTS

to clear from your mind

A RESTFUL MANTRA

to carry you to sleep

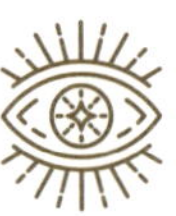

RUMINATING THOUGHTS

to clear from your mind

A RESTFUL MANTRA

to carry you to sleep

RUMINATING THOUGHTS

to clear from your mind

A RESTFUL MANTRA

to carry you to sleep

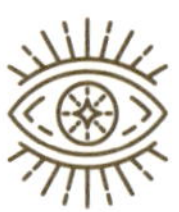

RUMINATING THOUGHTS

to clear from your mind

A RESTFUL MANTRA

to carry you to sleep

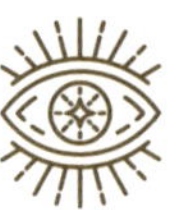

RUMINATING THOUGHTS

to clear from your mind

A RESTFUL MANTRA

to carry you to sleep

RUMINATING THOUGHTS

to clear from your mind

A RESTFUL MANTRA

to carry you to sleep

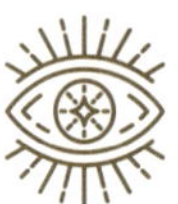

RUMINATING THOUGHTS

to clear from your mind

A RESTFUL MANTRA

to carry you to sleep

RUMINATING THOUGHTS

to clear from your mind

A RESTFUL MANTRA

to carry you to sleep

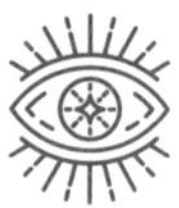

RUMINATING THOUGHTS

to clear from your mind

A RESTFUL MANTRA

to carry you to sleep

BRING AWARENESS TO YOUR BODY

"Sleep is the golden chain that ties health and our bodies together." —*Thomas Dekker*

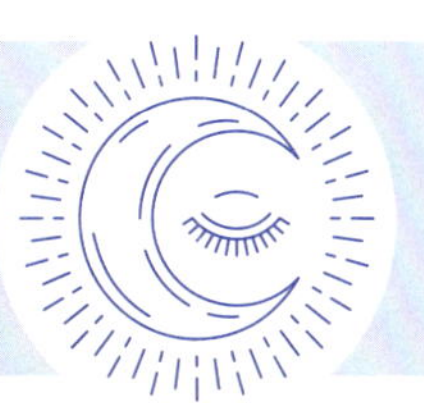

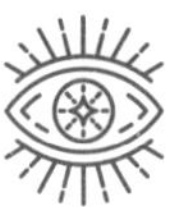

RUMINATING THOUGHTS

to clear from your mind

A RESTFUL MANTRA

to carry you to sleep

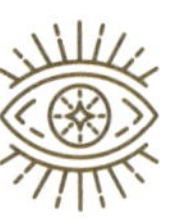

RUMINATING THOUGHTS

to clear from your mind

A RESTFUL MANTRA

to carry you to sleep

RUMINATING THOUGHTS

to clear from your mind

A RESTFUL MANTRA

to carry you to sleep

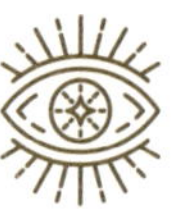

RUMINATING THOUGHTS

to clear from your mind

A RESTFUL MANTRA

to carry you to sleep

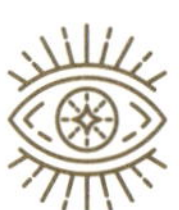

RUMINATING THOUGHTS

to clear from your mind

A RESTFUL MANTRA

to carry you to sleep

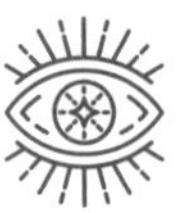

RUMINATING THOUGHTS

to clear from your mind

A RESTFUL MANTRA

to carry you to sleep

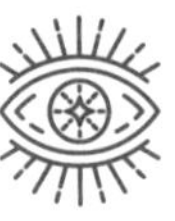

RUMINATING THOUGHTS

to clear from your mind

A RESTFUL MANTRA

to carry you to sleep

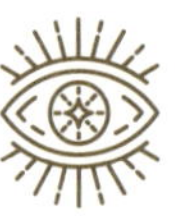

RUMINATING THOUGHTS

to clear from your mind

A RESTFUL MANTRA

to carry you to sleep

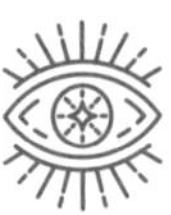

RUMINATING THOUGHTS

to clear from your mind

A RESTFUL MANTRA

to carry you to sleep

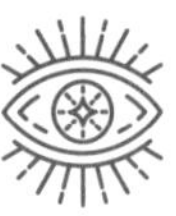

RUMINATING THOUGHTS

to clear from your mind

A RESTFUL MANTRA

to carry you to sleep

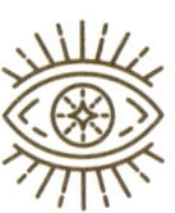

RUMINATING THOUGHTS

to clear from your mind

A RESTFUL MANTRA

to carry you to sleep

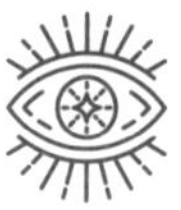

RUMINATING THOUGHTS

to clear from your mind

A RESTFUL MANTRA

to carry you to sleep

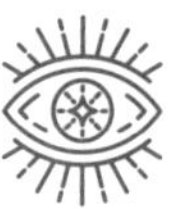

RUMINATING THOUGHTS

to clear from your mind

A RESTFUL MANTRA

to carry you to sleep

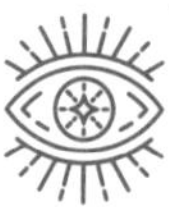

RUMINATING THOUGHTS

to clear from your mind

A RESTFUL MANTRA

to carry you to sleep

UNPLUG AND LET GO

"Turn off your mind, relax and float downstream." —John Lenon

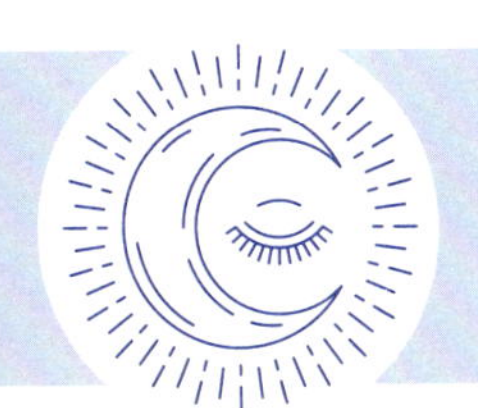

RUMINATING THOUGHTS

to clear from your mind

A RESTFUL MANTRA

to carry you to sleep

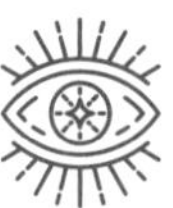

RUMINATING THOUGHTS

to clear from your mind

A RESTFUL MANTRA

to carry you to sleep

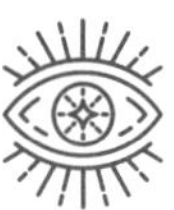

RUMINATING THOUGHTS

to clear from your mind

A RESTFUL MANTRA

to carry you to sleep

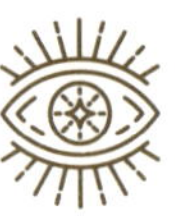

RUMINATING THOUGHTS

to clear from your mind

A RESTFUL MANTRA

to carry you to sleep

RUMINATING THOUGHTS

to clear from your mind

A RESTFUL MANTRA

to carry you to sleep

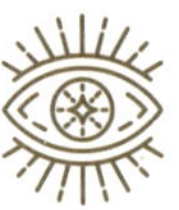

RUMINATING THOUGHTS

to clear from your mind

A RESTFUL MANTRA

to carry you to sleep

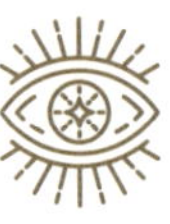

RUMINATING THOUGHTS

to clear from your mind

A RESTFUL MANTRA

to carry you to sleep

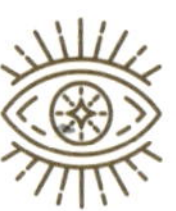

RUMINATING THOUGHTS

to clear from your mind

A RESTFUL MANTRA

to carry you to sleep

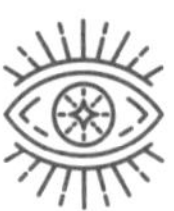

RUMINATING THOUGHTS

to clear from your mind

A RESTFUL MANTRA

to carry you to sleep

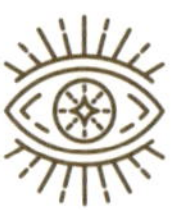

RUMINATING THOUGHTS

to clear from your mind

A RESTFUL MANTRA

to carry you to sleep

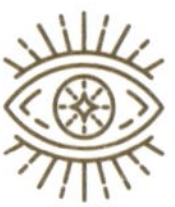

RUMINATING THOUGHTS

to clear from your mind

A RESTFUL MANTRA

to carry you to sleep

RUMINATING THOUGHTS

to clear from your mind

A RESTFUL MANTRA

to carry you to sleep

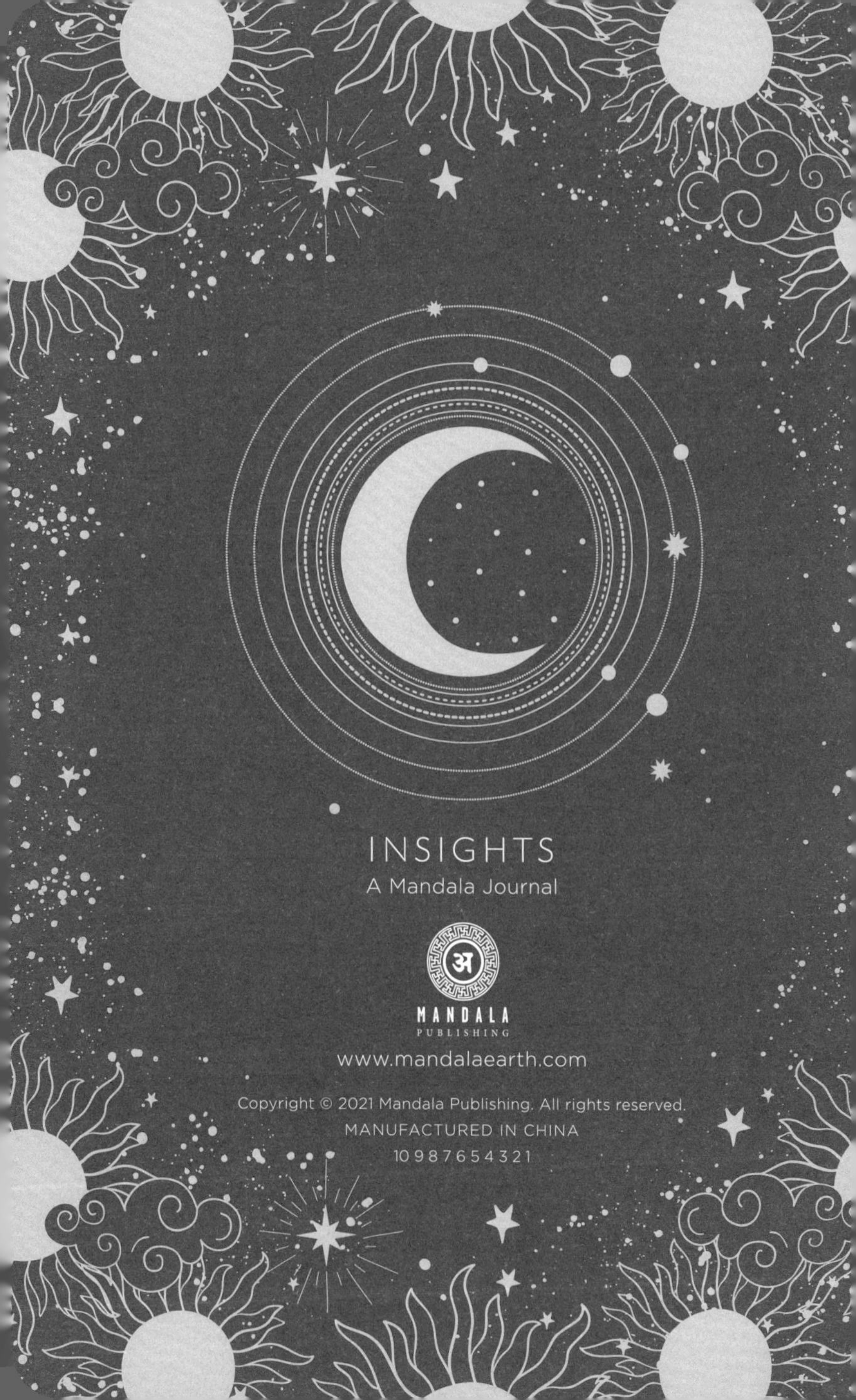

INSIGHTS

A Mandala Journal

www.mandalaearth.com

MANUFACTURED IN CHINA

10 9 8 7 6 5 4 3 2 1

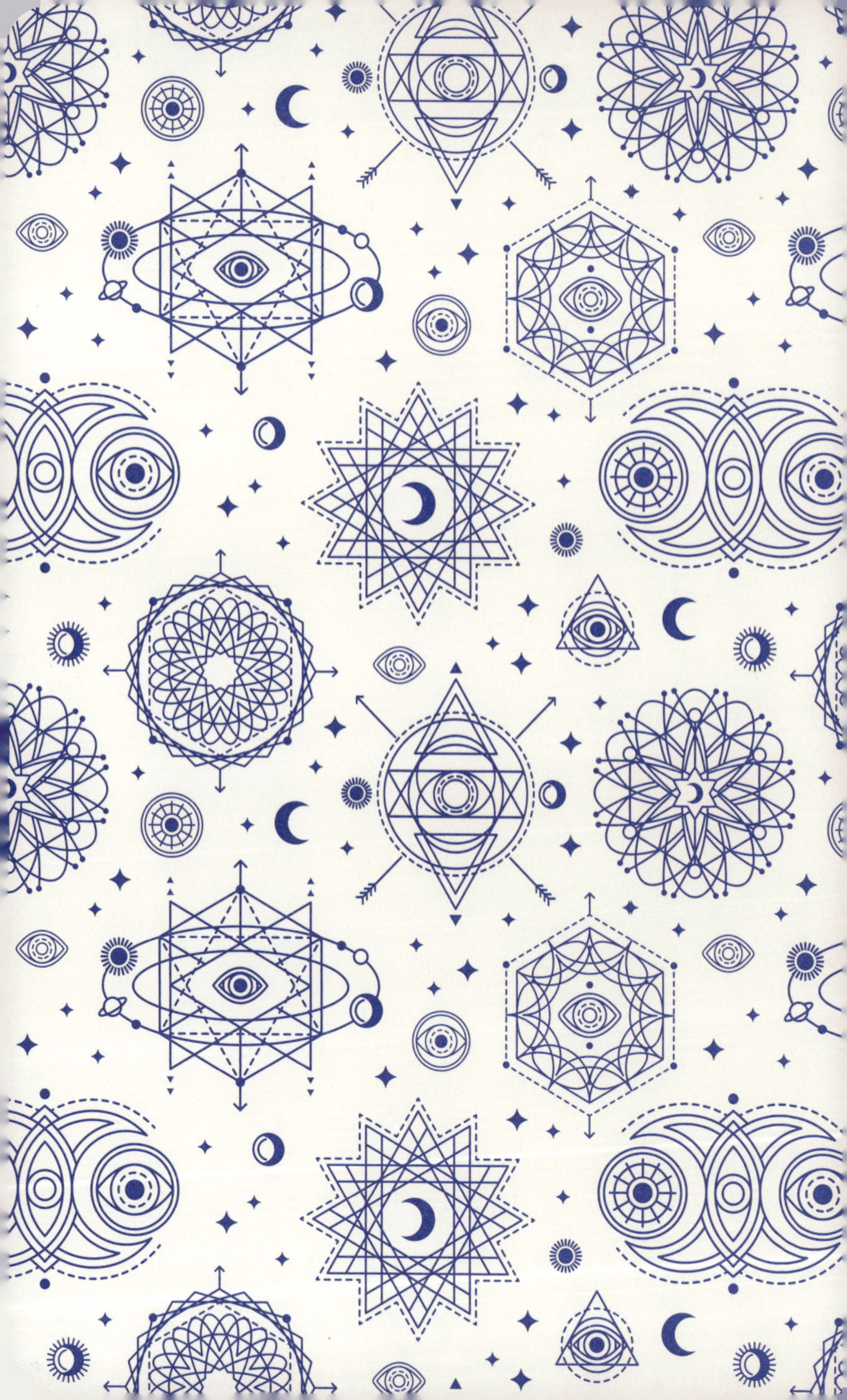